10 Steps to Loving Your Body

(No Matter What Size You Are)

Pat Ballard

Pearlsong Press
Nashville, TN

Pearlsong Press
P.O. Box 58065
Nashville, TN 37205
www.pearlsong.com
www.pearlsongpress.com

Book design by Zelda Pudding

The poem "live with intention" by mary anne radmacher is reprinted with permission from mary anne radmacher (www.maryanneradmacher.com).

Other books by Pat Ballard published by Pearlsong Press:
Dangerous Curves Ahead: Short Stories • *Wanted: One Groom* • *Nobody's Perfect* • *His Brother's Child* • *A Worthy Heir* • *Abigail's Revenge* • *The Best Man*

Quantity discounts are available to your business, institution or organization for reselling, gifts, fundraising or educational purposes, or incentives.
For more information contact
Pearlsong Press • P.O. Box 58065 • Nashville, TN 37205
615-356-5188 • sales@pearlsong.com

LIBRARY OF CONGRESS CATALOGING IN PUBLICATION DATA

Ballard, Pat (Patricia F.)
  10 steps to loving your body : (no matter what size you are) / Pat Ballard.
    p. cm.
  ISBN-13: 978-1-59719-014-5 (trade pbk. : alk. paper)
  ISBN-10: 1-59719-014-4 (trade pbk. : alk. paper)
  1. Body image in women. 2. Obesity in women—Psychological aspects. I. Title: Ten steps to loving your body. II. Title.
  BF697.5.B63B35 2008
  306.4'613—dc22
                        2008018107

What people have to say about Pat Ballard & her books

"Like so many women, Pat had been on and off fad diets since she was eleven. When she began to write, it seemed natural to her to make her heroines plus-size women. She has written a number of romance novels with Big Beautiful Heroines. The main characters are plus-size, but the message is for all women to love themselves as they are and stop trying to be something they were never meant to be."

Peggy Hoelne
Suite101.com

"Thank God, someone has the strength to be sane, and let a woman 'just be.' Someone can look the societal ideal in the eye and say 'no thanks, I'm valuable as I am.' Women are tired and overstressed from doing it all. The lengths we go to in order to 'fit the ideal body image' are undervalued. We need a collective 'enough already,' and to send out the message that who we are as individuals is worth enough. Thanks."

Jena Leonardo

"Ballard doesn't pull punches. She shows her heroines exhibiting ample will and tenacity to tell off those who would shame them into becoming something they aren't just to blend in with society's narrow-minded notions of beauty. There's no guilt in being a big, beautiful heroine in *Dangerous Curves Ahead*, and that is itself a formula for a classic happy ending."

C. Appel
Fearless Books

"Pat Ballard creates strong witty characters that pull you into the book, wanting to know more about their hopes and dreams."

Melissa Alvarez
About.com

"Finally, realistic heroines!...I'm not normally a romance novel reader (although I HAVE been known to read a few), but I was intrigued by the concept of realistic heroines....Ms. Ballard paints her characters with a vivid brush....This book proves that all women are beautiful, not just what Hollywood considers beautiful."

Rick Bentsen
author of *Dawn of a New Age (Gamma Strike)*
& *The Blademaster Chronicles*

"I think the idea that a large woman can be a heroine is long overdue, much like the idea that they are smart, witty, loving, healthy, sexy, passionate, and adventurous is long overdue!... Pat Ballard, thank you for trying to open the world's eyes and hearts!"

Jeffrey S. McCalla
of Houston, TX

"I love how your heroine was a strong woman who felt comfortable in her body no matter what size she was."

Brenda Condit

"It's so nice to read about a woman who isn't a 'perfect size six, and on the slender side' like so many of the other books I've read, or have her be a little heavy at the beginning of the book only to lose the 'excess' weight once she finds a man... I hope you start a new trend of books being written for real women!"

Tamara

Dedicated to Tim Segard,
formerly with iUniverse.com,
who gave me the idea to turn my
"10 Steps To Loving Your Body"
into a book.

Thanks, Tim.

STEP 1

Never stand in front of a mirror and think negative thoughts about yourself.

"People only see what they are prepared to see."

RALPH WALDO EMERSON

We've all done it. We stand in front of a mirror and look for the negative things about ourselves. Why do we do this? Somewhere in our young lives most of us learned, decided, or were taught that we're not good enough as we are. We're not pretty enough. We're not tall enough. We're not short enough. We're not thin enough. We're too thin, too short, too tall, too fat. We're— anything and everything *except* okay.

Why is it so hard for us to stand in front of that same mirror and look for the good things about ourselves? It's almost as if we have a built in self-disgustometer that won't allow us to see the good points that are just there waiting to be discovered, acknowledged and admired.

We all have good points. Go ahead. Find yours.

"Happiness is:

Looking in a mirror

and liking what you see."

ANONYMOUS

*"When I look in the mirror
I see the girl I was when I was growing up,
with braces, crooked teeth, a baby face
and a skinny body."*

HEATHER LOCKLEAR

How many of us are like Heather? She's a beautiful woman, but her eyes are trained to see herself at a time in her life when she obviously didn't like the way she looked.

Are we doing the same thing?

"You are always
a valuable,
worthwhile
human being—
not because anybody says so,
not because you're successful,
not because you make
a lot of money—
but because
you decide to believe it
and for no other reason."

WAYNE DYER

> *"When there is no enemy within,*
> *the enemies outside cannot hurt you."*

AFRICAN PROVERB

This is such a beautiful truth. When we learn to be at peace with ourselves, what others say and do to us doesn't hurt nearly as badly.

Sure, words hurt. I'll never try to make you believe that negative remarks don't hurt. But if we're acting as the "enemy within" and constantly bombarding ourselves with negative words of self-hate, the enemies outside are able to hurt us even more.

When we've accepted ourselves and learned to love the person we are, those words don't carry the same sting that they do if we *believe* they're true.

"I'd rather be able
to face myself in
the bathroom mirror
than be rich and famous."

ANI DIFRANCO

*"Accept yourself as you are.
Otherwise you will never see opportunity.
You will not feel free to move toward it;
you will feel you are not deserving."*

MAXWELL MALTZ

Hating oneself is dooming oneself to a life of bondage.

When a person hates the way she looks, the feeling is a constant companion. It affects every thought we have, every move we make. It burdens us down as if there were a huge backpack on our shoulders.

"When you feel good
about yourself,
others will feel good
about you, too."

JAKE STEINFELD

"It is of practical value to learn to like yourself. Since you must spend so much time with yourself you might as well get some satisfaction out of the relationship."

NORMAN VINCENT PEALE

I'll never forget the joy of learning to like myself.

After 23 years of dieting, I decided that I would stop my self-destructive dieting habits and eat as healthily as possible, exercise moderately when I had time or was so inclined, and learn to love the "me" that developed.

No, it wasn't an overnight success. But gradually, I was able to look into the mirror and see my good points. And gradually, I learned to like what I saw in the mirror.

I liked me!

"Dance
  as though
  no one
  is watching you.
Love
  as though you
  have never been
  hurt before.
Sing
  as though
  no one
  can hear you.
Live
  as though
  heaven is on earth."

Souza

Step forward

I will look for 10 positive things about myself—
and remember them every day.

Example:
    I have pretty eyes.
    (Feel free to use this as one of your own.)

1. _____

2. _____

3. _____

4. _____

5. _____

6. _____

7. _____

8. _____

9. _____

10. _____

10 STEPS TO LOVING YOUR BODY • PAT BALLARD

STEP 2

Never stand anywhere
and think negative thoughts
about yourself.

*"I will praise thee;
for I am fearfully [and] wonderfully made:
marvelous [are] thy works;
and [that] my soul knoweth right well."*

PSALMS 139:14 (KING JAMES VERSION)

King David acknowledged to God that he realized he was a work of art.

We are all wonderfully and marvelously made. Like King David, we should acknowledge this fact and give thanks for it.

"Our life is what
our thoughts make it."

Marcus Aurelius Antonius

*"While we have the gift of life,
it seems to me the only tragedy
is to allow part of us to die—
whether it is our spirit, our creativity,
or our glorious uniqueness."*

GILDA RADNER

"Our glorious uniqueness." I think that's the thing that most of us go through life not really appreciating.

We spend so much of our time trying to be like someone else. Trying to look like someone else. Trying to live someone else's life.

We not only let parts of ourselves die, as Gilda said, we actually spend time trying to *exterminate* parts of ourselves. Especially, our outer bodies.

Instead, we need to feed, nourish and cherish our bodies and learn to glory in our *individual uniqueness*.

"When you are
content to be
simply yourself
and don't
compare or compete,
everybody
will respect you."

LAO-TZU

*"Beware, as long as you live,
of judging people by appearances."*

JEAN DE LA FONTAINE

It has long been my contention that we're hard on ourselves because we're so hard on those around us.

It is so easy to point our fingers at those around us. Judging them by their appearances before we get to know them, then judging them maybe even worse *after* we get to know them.

Then we turn those thoughts inward and judge ourselves by the same standards. It's almost a two-edged sword.

When we learn to love ourselves, we will love those around us; but, also, when we learn to love and accept those around us, it makes it easier to love and accept ourselves.

"Remember always
that you have
not only the right
to be an individual,
but you have
an obligation
to be one."

ELEANOR ROOSEVELT

"The majority of people meet with failure because they lack the persistence to create new plans to take the place of failed plans."

MARK VICTOR HANSEN

Learning to stop putting yourself down, to stop finding fault with how you look, how your body is made, what size you are, etc., isn't enough. Along with stopping the stinking thinking about yourself, you've got to learn how to replace those negative thoughts with positive thoughts.

Every time you start to think a negative thought about yourself, just say *"NO!"* Say it out loud when possible.

Don't think that negative thought. Instead, replace the negative thought with a positive thought about yourself.

"I've got such fat thighs!" *NO!* "But I've got beautiful eyes." Or "I've got nice hair."

Don't just stop the negative. **Start the positive.**

"Begin challenging
   your own assumptions.
   Your assumptions
   are your windows
   on the world.
   Scrub them off
   every once in awhile,
   or the light
   won't come in."

ALAN ALDA

"Flatter me, and I may not believe you.
Criticize me, and I may not like you.
Ignore me, and I may not forgive you.
Encourage me, and I will not forget you."

WILLIAM ARTHUR WARD

To encourage means to inspire with courage, spirit, or hope; to spur on; to give help or patronage to. But is this something we just do to others? No. We have to encourage **ourselves**, also.

In fact, sometimes we're the only one around to encourage ourselves. So don't be afraid to tell yourself that you're "okay."

It always amazes me when I see a child respond to encouragement. When you say words of praise or encouragement to even very small children, they will literally start to strut! You can visually see the change in their facial expressions and they will walk with more confidence.

If we can make ourselves feel worse by talking down to ourselves, then it stands to reason that we can make ourselves feel better if we say encouraging words to ourselves.

live with intention.

walk to the edge.

listen hard.

practice wellness.

play with abandon.

l a u g h.

choose with no regret.

continue to learn.

appreciate your friends.

do what you love.

live as if this is all there is.

MARY ANNE RADMACHER

Step Forward

*I will look for 10 positive things to think about myself
when I'm in public.*

Example:
   I like the way I feel in this outfit.

1. _____

2. _____

3. _____

4. _____

5. _____

6. _____

7. _____

8. _____

9. _____

10. _____

10 Steps to Loving Your Body • Pat Ballard

STEP 3

Search carefully for
your good points and
when you have found them,
nourish them and build them
and cause them to grow daily.

*"It is as hard to see one's self
as to look backwards without turning around."*

HENRY DAVID THOREAU

Most of us have trained ourselves to see our very worst faults when we look into a mirror. We've trained our eyes to go to the spot or spots that we hate the most.

Now is the time to retrain our eyes. Find those good points. Embed them into your subconscious mind. Dwell on them until you really believe they're who you are.

"I finally realized
that being grateful
to my body
was key
to giving more love
to myself."

Oprah Winfrey

"A smile is an inexpensive way to improve your looks."

CHARLES GORDY

In fact, it costs nothing to smile, except maybe the effort to retrain some frown muscles. And a smile is one of the best points anyone can have.

A person can be the most beautiful being around, but if he or she wears a continual frown and has a terrible attitude, nobody cares how beautiful they are. So one of the first good features you need to recognize and start to build upon is your smile.

As Louis Armstrong says in one of his songs, "Smile, and the whole world smiles with you."

"People seldom notice old clothes
if you wear a big smile."

LEE MILDON

"I've never seen
a smiling face
that was not beautiful."

AUTHOR UNKNOWN

"Each individual woman's body demands to be accepted on its own terms."

GLORIA STEINEM

This is such a wonderful statement. This one sentence sums it up. And it is so true.

No matter how hard we fight it. No matter how much we starve ourselves, or how much we eat trying to gain weight, our bodies *know* what they want to look like. They're genetically programmed, so it doesn't matter how hard we fight it—they will fight back.

We should all print this quote and post it on our mirrors, in our bedrooms, in our purses, and any other place we can think of and read it over and over each day.

"Each body has its art..."

GWENDOLYN BROOKS

"Oh, darling, let your body in,
let it tie you in,
in comfort."

ANNE SEXTON
"Little Girl,
My String Bean,
My Lovely Woman"

What a joy it is when we become so at peace with our bodies that they are a comfort to us instead of "the enemy."

"People often say
that 'beauty is
in the eye of
the beholder,'
and I say
that the most
liberating thing
about beauty is
realizing that you
are the beholder.
This empowers us
to find beauty
in places where
others have not dared
to look, including
inside ourselves."

SALMA HAYEK

*"Women who set a low value on themselves
make life hard for all women."*

NELLIE McCLUNG

*"Until you value yourself
you will not value your time.
Until you value your time,
you will not do anything with it."*

M. SCOTT PECK

*"Think highly of yourself,
for the world takes you
at your own estimate."*

UNKNOWN

"People are like
stained-glass windows.
They sparkle and shine
when the sun is out,
but when the darkness sets in,
their true beauty is revealed only
if there is a light
from within."

ELIZABETH KÜBLER-ROSS

Step Forward

I will look for 10 good things about my body and try to develop them.

Example:
    I will try to smile more.

1. _____

2. _____

3. _____

4. _____

5. _____

6. _____

7. _____

8. _____

9. _____

10. _____

10 STEPS TO LOVING YOUR BODY • PAT BALLARD

STEP 4

Close your mind to any negative words, thoughts or actions that someone might send your way, and never let them enter your mind in any form or fashion. Never allow any person to say negative things to you or about you.

"To be nobody but yourself when the world is trying its best night and day to make you somebody else is to fight the hardest battle any human being will fight."

E.E. CUMMINGS

When a person says something negative to you, it's a good idea, if you can keep your calm and remember to do it, to just ask them why they would say something like that to another person.

Do they think they're that much better than you are? Or are they miserable and just trying to make you feel as badly as they do?

"A hurtful act is the transference to others of the degradation which we bear in ourselves."

SIMONE WEIL

"To let a sad thought
or a bad one
get into your mind
is as dangerous as letting
a scarlet-fever germ
get into your body.
If you let it stay there
after it has got in,
you may never
get over it
as long as
you live."

FRANCES HODGSON BURNETT

"It took a long time not to judge myself through other people's eyes."

Unknown

When I was still on the dieting roller coaster and would be on my way "back up" after having lost weight, I would put myself down when in the presence of someone I hadn't seen in a while. My theory was that I *knew* they were thinking that I was regaining the weight I'd lost, so I might as well point out the obvious to them so they would know that I was aware of how really bad I looked.

DO NOT DO THIS!

I don't care if you have to bite your tongue until it looks like a perforated "tear along this line" sign. **DO NOT PUT YOURSELF DOWN TO OTHERS!**

It just opens up the door for them to join you in your self-degradation.

"Count him not
among your friends
who will retail
your privacies
to the world."

Publilus Syrus

"He that respects himself is safe from others;
he wears a coat of mail that none can pierce."

HENRY WADSWORTH LONGFELLOW

Once we learn to respect ourselves, we won't allow someone to demean us.

And the more we learn to respect ourselves, the easier it will be to stop someone when they say something negative to us: "I know you mean well, but please don't say those things to me."

"I prefer to be true to myself,
even at the hazard of incurring the ridicule of others,
rather than to be false,
and to incur my own abhorrence."

FREDERICK DOUGLASS

"They cannot take away
our self-respect
if we do not
give it to them."

MAHATMA GANDHI

*"To free us from the expectations of others,
to give us back to ourselves—
there lies the great, singular power
of self-respect."*

JOAN DIDION

We can't please everyone in our lives. We all know it, but, for some reason we keep trying to please those who sling the nastiest remarks our way. It's time to stop doing this. It's time to free ourselves from the expectations of others and to take back "ourselves."

"Mother, I can't be the svelte daughter that you want me to be. But I'm *me*. And I'm your daughter, so love me."

"Friend, I know you think you're looking out for my health, but you don't have all the facts. So just be my friend and stop trying to be my advisor."

Claim yourself. Claim that one-of-a-kind work of art that you are.

Claim it and respect it and be happy with it.

"If I
despised myself,
it would be
no compensation
if everyone
saluted me,
and
if I
respect myself,
it does not
trouble me
if others
hold me lightly."

MAX NORDAU

"A successful person is one who can lay a firm foundation with the bricks that others throw at him or her."

DAVID BRINKLEY

"It ain't what they call you, it's what you answer to."

W.C. FIELDS

At first glance, the saying by W.C. Fields is just humorous. But let's look at this quote a little deeper, because there's a lot of truth in it.

If you're constantly putting yourself down, belittling yourself and thinking negative thoughts about yourself, when someone else does the same thing you're going to think they're right. You won't be as offended by their words because you'll agree with them.

So, in essence, you'll answer to what they call you. But once you stop allowing these negatives into your life, then you won't "answer" to negative things that are said to and about you.

"A man can stand a lot as long as he can stand himself."

AXEL MUNTHE

"If you want
to be respected by others
the great thing is
to respect yourself.
Only by that,
only by self-respect
will you compel others
to respect you."

Fyodor Dostoyevsky

STEP FORWARD

I will look for 10 ways to deal with negative words
or actions that I get from others.

Example:
    "Excuse me? I don't appreciate you saying that to me."

1. _____

2. _____

3. _____

4. _____

5. _____

6. _____

7. _____

8. _____

9. _____

10. _____

10 Steps to Loving Your Body • Pat Ballard

STEP 5

Always conduct yourself
in an honorable fashion
and don't allow your mouth
to appear larger than your body.

*"We live by encouragement and die without it—
slowly, sadly, angrily."*

CELESTE HOLM

I've witnessed a lot of plus-sized women with a loud, "in-your-face" type of attitude. I've never asked one of them why they conduct themselves in this manner, but I've wondered if they're insecure about their size and think that if they make enough "mouth-noise" nobody will notice their bodies.

I'm only speculating here, and truly don't want to impute motive when there is none, but in these women I've also sensed the insecure child inside. I can almost feel their pain. Their anger.

It's as if they're fighting back at all those around them because they're hurting so badly.

"We run away
all the time
to avoid
coming face to face
with ourselves."

AUTHOR UNKNOWN

*"We all have to go through the awkward stage
of any newly acquired behavior....
There will be more firsts that we will encounter
in which we will feel awkward for a while,
until we get the hang of it....
Any thing you want to learn,
you are going to be awkward at it at first.
Give yourself permission to be a beginner,
a learner."*

JACK CANFIELD & MARK V. HANSON
The Aladdin Factor

When you're programmed to think a certain way, to act a certain way, and then you try to change that way of thinking and acting, you'll probably feel like you're literally stepping outside of yourself. You'll feel like the quote above suggests. You might even feel "silly" and/or very conspicuous.

But breaking the habit of thinking negative thoughts or acting in a negative way is just like breaking any other habit. It will be hard at first, but soon the new way of thinking and acting will become habit and will be as natural as what you're trying to stop doing.

"An optimist
is a person
who undertakes a
seemingly impossible task
in a spirit of
immeasurable enthusiasm,
unbounded determination,
unbelievable excitement,
indestructible confidence,
uncompromising thoroughness,
and indefatigable
persistence...
with understandable
success."

WILLIAM ARTHUR WARD

"I believe a person should be grateful
for his life and his opportunity
to live and learn and grow
in a climate where he is free to choose
what he will do,
how much he will do,
and how far he'll go
with the time and talents
he's been given."

EARL NIGHTINGALE

How can we feel grateful for our lives if we're constantly miserable about how we look?

If we're wasting our brainpower on obsessing over the fact that we don't look like someone who just stepped off of a page of the latest magazine, then we're not grateful for our own lives. For our own looks. For the individual beings that we are.

"A human being
is a part of a whole,
called by us 'universe,'
a part limited in time
and space. He experiences
himself, his thoughts and
feelings as something separated
from the rest...a kind of
optical delusion of his
consciousness. This delusion is
a kind of prison for us,
restricting us to our personal
desires and to affection for
a few persons nearest to us.
Our task must be to free
ourselves from this prison
by widening our circle of
compassion to embrace all
living creatures and
the whole of nature
in its beauty."

ALBERT EINSTEIN

*"It's surprising how many persons go through life
without ever recognizing that their feelings
toward other people are largely determined
by their feelings toward themselves,
and if you're not comfortable within yourself,
you can't be comfortable with others."*

SIDNEY J. HARRIS

*"Other people's opinion of you
does not have to become your reality."*

LES BROWN

*"It took me a long time not to judge myself
through someone else's eyes."*

SALLY FIELD

"If only
    you could sense
    how important you are
    to the lives of
    those you meet;
    how important you can be
    to people you may never
    even dream of.
    There is
    something of yourself
    that you leave
    at every meeting
    with another person."

FRED ROGERS

*"Human beings, by changing
the inner attitudes of their minds,
can change the outer aspects of their lives."*

WILLIAM JAMES

How very true. If we change the way we think about ourselves, then we can change the way we feel about ourselves. The way we see ourselves. Our lives will start to *be* different because we will *see* them differently.

*"If you change the way you look at things,
the things you look at change."*

WAYNE DYER

"At bottom
every man knows well enough
that he is a unique being,
only once on this earth;
and by no extraordinary chance
will such a marvelously
picturesque piece
of diversity in unity
as he is, ever be put together
a second time."

FRIEDRICH WILHELM NIETZSCHE

Step Forward

I will look for 10 ways in which I may be trying
to "hide" my body behind my words.

Example:
 The next time I see someone staring at me, I won't
 think or say, "What are you looking at?" I'll just
 assume they *like* what they see.

1. _____

2. _____

3. _____

4. _____

5. _____

6. _____

7. _____

8. _____

9. _____

10. _____

10 Steps to Loving Your Body • Pat Ballard

Step 6

Always do your best
to look like you care
about yourself,
as no one respects a slob,
no matter what size
that slob might be.

*"Know, first, who you are;
and then adorn yourself accordingly."*

Epictetus

I enjoy getting up every day and dressing as if I'm going to meet a friend for lunch, whether I'm going anywhere or not. I put on my makeup, fix my hair and dress in a manner that if the phone rings and I get a call to "let's do lunch," all I have to do is pick up my purse and walk out the door.

But that's not the real reason I dress like this every day. I do it for myself. When I lounge around all day in sloppy clothes, then I feel sloppy all day. It truly affects my thought patterns. I know I *look* sloppy, so I *feel* sloppy. I don't feel as productive. I feel as if I'm "coming down with something," or in some way on the verge of being sick.

But this is me. This is who I am. So I'm not suggesting that everyone *must* get up every morning and dress for an outing. But I challenge you to try it and see if you don't feel a lot better throughout your day. You might even have more energy.

I'm not suggesting that you *must* put on your makeup, comb your hair and look "nice" when you go out. But I am suggesting that you're not doing yourself any favors when you leave your house looking like you've been working in your flower garden all day. Or looking like you just got out of bed. When you're dressed like that it appears that you don't respect yourself, so others won't respect you as much, either.

As I write this, I'm hearing a multitude of voices yelling at me, "But this is the way I feel comfortable! I don't want to have to do all that 'stuff' just to look a certain way." And that's fine, if that's who you are. If that's who you want to be.

But I dare you just to try the other way for two weeks and see if you feel the difference.

"Seldom do people
discern eloquence
under a threadbare cloak."

JUVENAL

"What a strange power there is in clothing."

Isaac Bashevis Singer

*"Young children, even, are susceptible to the effect of clothes.
A child dressed in dingy rags slouches and shrinks
when observed; the same child adorned
with a new ribbon or a pair of new shoes
will brighten and grow confident.
One day in a very poor district of the city
a test was made to verify this theory.
A dirty, ragged little girl was found
and over her soiled clothes a new, clean dress was hung.
Immediately she was changed from a broken-spirited
listless child to a saucy and rather impudent little creature.
Then all her clothes were removed; she was put in a tub,
and given the most thorough scrubbing of her young life;
her hair was shampooed, her nails manicured,
and she was dressed in a complete outfit
of clean, pretty clothes. The transformation in her manner
was startling. Gone was every trace of the gamin impudence.
She became, through her unconscious reaction
to cleanliness and clothes,
a self-respecting and respectful little woman."*

J. C. Fluegel
The Psychology of Clothes

"Clothes make the man.
Naked people have
little or no influence
on society."

MARK TWAIN

*"There is only one corner of the universe
you can be certain of improving,
and that's your own self."*

ALDOUS LEONARD HUXLEY

Most of the time, "self" is the last place we try to improve. I think some folks believe that if they keep pointing their finger away from themselves, then others won't notice them.

But as the old saying goes, "When you're pointing at someone else, three fingers are always pointing back at you."

"To be a fashionable woman
   is to know yourself,
   know what you represent,
   and know what
   works for you.
  To be 'in fashion'
   could be a disaster
   on 90 percent of women.
   You are not
   a page out of Vogue."

AUTHOR UNKNOWN

"There is new strength,
repose of mind,
and inspiration
in fresh apparel."

ELLA WHEELER WILCOX

We've all noticed how a new garment that we really like will lift our spirits. It makes us smile. It makes us feel good about how we look. We greet the world with a different expression on our faces, and the world looks back at us and smiles.

"Exuberance is beauty."

WILLIAM BLAKE

*"I have lived in this body all my life
and know it better than any fashion designer;
I am only willing to purchase the item which becomes me
and to wear that which enhances my image of myself
to myself."*

MAYA ANGELOU

This is what should be our goal. To wear the things that "become us," and that enhance the image that we have of ourselves.

But first, we have to learn to have a *good* image of ourselves. And wearing the correct clothes and makeup can create and enhance that image.

"The worst loneliness
is not to be comfortable
with yourself."

MARK TWAIN

Step Forward

*I will look for 10 ways to show that
I care about my body.*

Example:

I will comb my hair before I go shopping.

1. _____

2. _____

3. _____

4. _____

5. _____

6. _____

7. _____

8. _____

9. _____

10. _____

10 Steps to Loving Your Body • Pat Ballard

Step 7

Learn what your best colors are,
what your best hair style is,
and what your best clothes style is,
and never leave your house
without being dressed accordingly.

I used to think that if a person truly wants to improve his or her style, there is no reason for them not to be able to. But I've had to change my dogmatic opinion on this subject.

My husband, Joe, and I watch a show on Friday night titled *What Not To Wear,* with Stacy London and Clinton Kelly. This is the U.S. version that airs on TLC—The Learning Channel. The concept of the show is that friends, family and/or coworkers nominate someone for the show. If the nominee is chosen, they get $5,000 and get to go to New York City, where Stacey and Clinton help them find their best style for clothes, hair and makeup.

One of the things I appreciate about this show is that "losing weight" is never an option or suggestion for looking better. Stacey and Clinton will help the people learn to dress the bodies that they're in right now.

What has surprised and amazed me in watching this

show is that there are people, usually women, who honestly do not know how to shop for themselves, or in some cases, just hate to shop so they don't bother. And most of the time when these people go through the routine with Stacey and Kelly, they are amazed at how beautiful they wind up looking. They come away with a new or renewed self-esteem that they didn't have before.

If a person truly wants to improve the way she looks, there are ways to learn how to do this.

1. Is there someone you know whom you admire for the way they look, dress, carry themselves, etc.? Ask them for advice. Ask them to go shopping with you. Don't be ashamed to ask for help.

2. Buy magazines for the clothing tips, makeup tips, etc.—NOT for the diet tips.

3. Many department stores offer free facials. Treat yourself to a facial and learn what your best makeup colors are.

4. Watch *What Not To Wear* and similar shows.

5. Order clothing catalogs so you can study the styles, jewelry and makeup the models have on. You can learn a lot just from studying these photos.

If you live in an area where clothes in your size aren't available, you can go online to your favorite search engine and type in something like "clothes for size [your size here]" or "catalogs for size [your size here]." This should give you many options to either order online or request mail-order catalogs. A lot of the catalogs will be free.

Tip: Open your hand and look at the color of your palm and the muscle part of your thumb. Cool-toned skin has blue and pink undertones, while warm-toned skin has peach or gold undertones. Most makeup will indicate if it's "cool" or "warm."

You can also choose your clothes colors by this method. There are a lot of websites that teach how to do this. Just type something like "how to choose what color to wear" into your favorite search engine and several helpful websites will come up.

And you can always ask a salesperson in a department store to help you.

"Hair style is
the final tip-off
whether or not a woman
really knows herself."

Hubert de Givenchy

*"You can take no credit for beauty at sixteen.
But if you are beautiful at sixty,
it will be your soul's own doing."*

Actually, for most of us, this is true at any age. Most of us don't just get out of bed in the morning looking beautiful. And most of us hate the few who do! It doesn't take a lot of work or time to get up in the morning and comb our hair, put on a little makeup and some clothes. It only takes me five minutes to put on my makeup.

*"The greatest discovery of my generation
is that a human being can alter his life
by altering his attitudes."*

WILLIAM JAMES

"All changes,
even the most longed for,
have their melancholy;
for what we leave
behind us is
a part of ourselves;
we must die to one life
before we can
enter another."

ANATOLE FRANCE

*"We awaken in others
the same attitude of mind
we hold toward them."*

ELBERT HUBBARD

I would like to go a little further with this thought and suggest that we do the same with ourselves. We awaken in ourselves the same attitude of mind that we hold toward ourselves.

*"The only difference between a rut and a grave
is their dimensions."*

ELLEN GLASGOW

"Just around the corner
   in every woman's mind—
   is a lovely dress,
   a wonderful suit,
   or entire costume
   which will make
   an enchanting new creature
   of her."

WILHELA CUSHMAN

"Carelessness in dressing is moral suicide."

HONORÉ DE BALZAC

I f you don't think dressing a certain way affects you, ask yourself how you would react to the following scenarios.

SAY YOU HAVE CHILDREN and you've put an ad in the newspaper for a babysitter. Two female candidates (teenagers) show up at your door.

One of them is featuring the popular "Gothic" look. Dyed black, dirty hair, eye makeup so dark it looks like a month-long hangover, black lipstick, crossbones as a necklace, skull rings on all 10 fingers, a T-shirt that says "Show No Fear," and grungy jeans with big holes in them.

Now this person may be as good as gold and just trying to look like the latest style, but you don't really know that unless you know them personally.

The other girl has shiny, clean hair, tasteful makeup,

clean clothes, shoes that actually match, a few rings, but clean fingernails.

Tell me, honestly: Which one of these people would you want to take care of your children, given they were otherwise similar in their qualifications?

Now, LET'S DO ONE MORE scenario. You have the responsibility of interviewing someone for the position of receptionist for the company where you work. Two candidates come in. They're both women.

One of them looks as if she's just stepped out of the fashion pages of the latest women's magazine. Hair, clothes, shoes, nails, makeup are all done to perfection. She doesn't have quite all the qualifications that you need for the job, but you can tell that she would be a quick learner.

The other woman is in a faded jogging suit and tennis shoes. She looks like she was cleaning house and remembered she had an appointment for the interview.

Her hair is long and stringy and not too clean. She doesn't appear to have on any makeup and her nails have the faintest tint of darkness under them, so you think that she might have been working in her garden before she dashed to the interview. She sees you casually looking her over and quickly assures you that she "doesn't like to dress up. This is much more comfortable" to her.

Her qualifications for the job are actually better than the other woman.

Which one of these women would you want representing your company?

DRESSING CASUALLY and dressing sloppily are two entirely different things. Jeans or slacks with a knit top or button shirt, etc., are casual. Jogging pants and a T-shirt that says

"I'm Bubba's" are sloppy—I don't care if you're a size 0 or a size 50.

Again, if you want to be seen in public looking sloppy, that's your choice. I'm just saying...

"Clothes are
 never a frivolity:
 They always
 mean something."

JAMES LAVER

*"It's not who you are that holds you back,
it's who you think you're not."*

AUTHOR UNKNOWN

*"It's hard to fight an enemy
who has outposts in your head."*

SALLY KEMPTON

*"When the grass looks greener
on the other side of the fence,
it may be that they take better care of it there."*

CECIL SELIG

"I am convinced that attitude
is the key to success or failure
in almost any of
life's endeavors.
Your attitude—
your perspective, your outlook,
how you feel about yourself,
how you feel about
other people—determines
your priorities, your actions,
your values. Your attitude
determines how you interact
with other people and
how you interact with yourself."

CAROLYN WARNER

STEP FORWARD

I will look for 10 "beauty tips"
that will enhance my self-image.

Example:
    I will ask someone to help me find my best colors.

1. _____

2. _____

3. _____

4. _____

5. _____

6. _____

7. _____

8. _____

9. _____

10. _____

10 STEPS TO LOVING YOUR BODY • PAT BALLARD

Step 8

Always, and without fail, smile and simply say, "Thank you" when you receive a compliment. Never think or say that the compliment isn't true.

Why is it so hard for some of us to accept a compliment?

We go shopping and find something—a garment, shoes, purse, whatever—that we really like. We purchase it. We're excited to own it. Yet when someone compliments us on it, we start to make excuses as to why the item is "less than."

Why? Do we not think we're worthy of the item? Do we think we're not deserving of the compliment? Why?

The same goes with compliments about our looks. For a lot of people it's just plain uncomfortable to receive a compliment on anything. Yet we all need compliments. Compliments just make us *feel* better.

So please, from now on, when you receive a compliment *make* yourself simply smile and say, "Thank you!" If the compliment is about an item, it's even okay to say that you like it, too.

> *"Gratitude is the sign of noble souls."*
>
> Aesop's Fables

"I can live
 for two months
 on a good compliment."

MARK TWAIN

*"Other men it is said have seen angels,
but I have seen thee
and thou art enough."*

GEORGE MOORE

I want us to role-play, here. I want you to stop, right now, and pretend that someone has just said the above words to you.

Let's make it even more fun. Pretend that your greatest fantasy has said these words to you. Think of an actor or person in real life who makes you swoon. Now, pretend that person has called your name and said, "Other men it is said have seen angels, but I have seen you and you are enough."

Now, all *you* have to do is just smile and say, "Thank you!"

Don't say or think something like, "Well, you must need glasses, because it's obvious you have vision problems." In my former stinking-thinking life, I've actually used those words. DON'T DO THIS!

If you'll start practicing accepting compliments and put it into action, in a very short time it will become second nature. It will become easy.

And the bottom line is that when someone gives you a compliment, it's actually an insult to throw it back in his or her face. If they're sincere about their compliments, then it's rude to tell them that their opinions are wrong.

"The happiness of life
  is made up of
  minute fractions—
  the little,
  soon forgotten charities
  of a kiss or a smile,
  a kind look or
  heartfelt compliment."

Samuel Taylor Coleridge

"Too often we underestimate the power of a touch,
a smile, a kind word, a listening ear,
an honest compliment, or the smallest act of caring,
all of which have the potential
to turn a life around."

LEO BUSCAGLIA

B y the same token, too often we underestimate the importance that someone's heartfelt compliment can be to our own self-esteem. By denying or saying that the compliment isn't true, we're telling ourselves that we aren't praiseworthy and aren't "allowed" to feel good about our bodies.

"Everybody
likes a compliment."

ABRAHAM LINCOLN

"Pleasant words [are as] an honeycomb,
sweet to the soul,
and health to the bones."

Proverbs 16:24

"When you cannot get a compliment in any other way
pay yourself one."

Mark Twain

"A compliment is verbal sunshine."

Robert Orben

"A compliment is a gift,
not to be thrown away
carelessly,
unless you want
to hurt the giver."

ELEANOR HAMILTON

"I can no other answer make, but, thanks, and thanks."

WILLIAM SHAKESPEARE

And nothing more is needed.

"Silent gratitude isn't much use to anyone."

G.B. STERN

*"Every time we remember to say 'thank you,'
we experience nothing less than heaven on earth."*

SARAH BAN BREATHNACH

"Make it a habit
to tell people thank you.
To express your appreciation,
sincerely and without
the expectation
of anything in return.
Truly appreciate
those around you,
and you'll soon find
many others around you.
Truly appreciate life,
and you'll find
that you have more of it."

RALPH MARSTON

Step Forward

I will look for 10 ways to stop putting myself down.

Example:
   I will not say things like, "I'm so fat I look like the Goodyear Blimp."

1. _____

2. _____

3. _____

4. _____

5. _____

6. _____

7. _____

8. _____

9. _____

10. _____

10 Steps to Loving Your Body • Pat Ballard

STEP 9

Stop apologizing about your size,
and expect the world
and everyone in it
to accept you, respect you,
and be happy with you
just the way you are.

During the years of my yo-yo dieting, when I would be on my way "back up," as I called it, I was so conscious of the fact that I had gained weight that I assumed that was on *everybody* else's mind. So I always felt compelled to state what I thought was the "obvious." "I know I'm fat, but I'm going on a diet soon." And most of the time the person I was talking to would assure me that they hadn't even thought about my weight. Of course, at the time I didn't believe them. I had figured I'd speak up and let them know I knew I was fat.

DO NOT DO THIS!!!

Don't ever say things like, "I know I'm fat, but—" Or, "My butt's so big I can't get through the door."

Don't mention weight. If someone you're with brings up the topic of weight, handle it in a professional, impersonal manner, as if they're not talking to or about you at all. Then, if they do bring it to you personally, tell them that

"This is who I am, and if you don't like me just like I am, you're the one with a problem."

There is a lot of power in doing this. I was at a party once where there was an older woman who had ranted and raved about how beautiful she thought I was until it was beginning to be a little embarrassing to me.

Then, after she'd had a few glasses of wine, she said to me, "You're just so beautiful! But I'll bet if you lost 50 lbs, you'd be a knockout!"

I leaned down real close to her, so that only she could hear me, and whispered, "Love me just like I am or leave me alone!"

She didn't say anything else about me losing weight. And I felt really good!

"We have to learn to be our own best friends because we fall too easily into the trap of being our own worst enemies."

RODERICK THORP

"Never make a defense
or an apology
until you are accused."

KING CHARLES I

*"If you really put a small value upon yourself,
rest assured that the world will not raise your price."*

AUTHOR UNKNOWN

*"Of all our infirmities,
the most savage is to despise our being."*

MICHEL DE MONTAIGNE

*"I've been on a diet for two weeks
and all I've lost is fourteen days."*

TOTIE FIELDS

"Curve:
The loveliest distance
between two points."

Mae West

> *"Can you imagine a world without men?*
> *No crime and lots of happy fat women."*

NICOLE HOLLANDER

Actually, I have to disagree with this quote. At first glance, it sounds so true. But it has been my contention for a very long time that women dress *for women*. Not for the men in their lives. Not for themselves. And in a lot of cases, not even for success.

I'll be really brave and venture to say that the majority of women diet, exercise, and dress to impress other women. Their friends, their coworkers, and even women they don't really like! As women, we continually compare ourselves with other women.

When I was in the dieting world, I told myself "No man would like me as a fat woman." And I've heard other women say the same thing. But as I learned to love my body, and as I gained confidence in that body, I was in for a great surprise. I found out that *a lot* of men *really* like full-figured women.

I've had men tell me they wished their wives would stop dieting; that they liked her better with a little "meat on her bones."

One woman I worked with, who I'm pretty sure had anorexia, told me that her husband hated that she kept her body slim. She showed me photos of herself when she was much larger and said he liked her better at that size. She also told me that he said to her, "Oh well, I have my memories."

Yet she continued to diet and keep her body the way she thought looked good to her and her friends.

So I'd like to rewrite the above quote:

"Can you imagine a world without diets?
Lots of happy fat women,
and lots of even happier men."

PAT BALLARD

"The rarest thing
in the world
is a woman who is pleased
with photographs
of herself."

ELIZABETH METCALF

> *"Take care of your body.*
> *It's the only place you have to live."*

> Jim Rohn

A starved body is a weak body. When I was on my last weight-loss diet, I kept asking myself, "Why am I doing this to me? Why am I starving myself to look like some society says I'm supposed to look? If the average housewife needs 2,000 calories a day (the amount of calories that most standards go by) to perform her daily chores, then why should I be required to live on half that?"

People who keep themselves starved to lose weight are losing more than weight. They're losing out on any quality of life. They're going through life on half the fuel they need to feed their bodies, which fuel their brains. Their inherent power is being stolen from them simply because they're too hungry to operate at full capacity.

I know—I've been there.

> *"If the body be feeble,*
> *the mind will not be strong."*

> Thomas Jefferson

> *"Hunger:*
> *One of the few cravings*
> *that cannot be appeased*
> *with another solution."*

> Irwin Van Grove

"When we lose twenty pounds...
we may be losing
the twenty best pounds
we have!
We may be losing the pounds
that contain our genius,
our humanity,
our love and honesty."

WOODY ALLEN

"I use the word 'fat.'
I use that word because that's what people are:
They're fat. They're not bulky;
they're not large, chunky, hefty or plump.
And they're not big-boned. Dinosaurs were big-boned.
These people are not overweight:
This term somehow implies there is some correct weight.
There is no correct weight.
Heavy is also a misleading term.
An aircraft carrier is heavy; it's not fat.
Only people are fat,
and that's what fat people are!
They're fat!"

GEORGE CARLIN

In his own comedic way, I think George Carlin sums it up pretty well with these words.

I use the word "fat" a lot. Fat is not a four-letter word. It's not a "bad" word. When describing a person, it's just an adjective, like "tall," "short," and "slim." Fat.

"The leading cause of death among fashion models
is falling through street grates."

DAVE BARRY

"Our own physical body
possesses a wisdom
which we who inhabit the body
lack. We give it orders
which make no sense."

HENRY MILLER

Step Forward

I will look for 10 ways to stop apologizing for my size, because this opens the door for others to disrespect me.

Example:
I will not say things like "I know I need to go on a diet, but…"

1. _____

2. _____

3. _____

4. _____

5. _____

6. _____

7. _____

8. _____

9. _____

10. _____

10 Steps to Loving Your Body • Pat Ballard

Step 10

Most of all, you have to love yourself. When you love yourself, others will love you and respond to you in the exact manner as you feel about yourself.

"Love yourself first and everything else falls into line. You really have to love yourself to get anything done in this world."

LUCILLE BALL

We're admonished in nine different verses of the King James Version of the Bible to love our neighbors as *ourselves*. **We're expected to love ourselves.**

"For all the law is fulfilled in one word, [even] in this; Thou shalt love thy neighbour as thyself."

GALATIANS 5:14

"For no man ever yet hated his own flesh; but nourisheth [the Greek word means to nourish, support, feed, to give suck, to fatten, to bring up, nurture] *and cherisheth* [the Greek word means to warm, keep warm, to cherish with tender love, to foster with tender care] *it, even as the Lord the church."*

EPHESIANS 5:29

"To wish you were
   someone else
   is to waste
   the person you are."

ANONYMOUS

*"Always be a first-rate version of yourself,
instead of a second-rate version of somebody else."*

JUDY GARLAND

This is a very hard lesson to learn when we're bombarded daily with messages from every direction that we need to be anything *but* ourselves.
If my "self" is too fat, then I need to change it.
If my "self" is too thin, then I need to change it.
If my "self" is too short or tall, then I need to change it.
NO!
As Judy suggests, we need to be a first rate version of *this* "self" and love it just like it is.

"It takes courage
to grow up
and become
who you really are."

E.E. CUMMINGS

"Never be bullied into silence.
Never allow yourself to be made a victim.
Accept no one's definition of your life;
define yourself."

HARVEY FIERSTEIN

There will always be some well-meaning person who will try to tell you that you're too fat, too thin, or too "something."

It doesn't matter if it's your mate, your parent, your sibling, your best friend or a total stranger. If anyone—*anyone*—tells you that you aren't "good enough" because you look a certain way, don't listen to him or her.

And if you can do it, have a talk with that person and let it be known that you're happy with who you are and they will have to accept you just as you are, because you have.

"Let the world
 know you as you are,
 not as you think you should be,
 because sooner or later,
 if you are posing,
 you will forget the pose,
 and then where are you?"

FANNY BRICE

"There is just one life for each of us: our own."

EURIPIDES

What a sad waste it would be if we reach the end of our days and realize that we have never actually appreciated who we really are. To know that we spent our lives trying to live a life that someone else mapped out for us.

By then it will be too late to go back and live our own lives. What a sad, sad thing to realize that we'll take our "what could have been" to the grave.

"If God
had wanted me otherwise,
He would have created me
otherwise."

JOHANN VON GOETHE

*"All my life I had been looking for something,
and everywhere I turned someone tried to tell me
what it was. I accepted their answers too,
though they were often in contradiction
and even self-contradictory. I was naïve.
I was looking for myself and asking everyone except myself
questions which I, and only I, could answer.
It took me a long time and much painful boomeranging
of my expectations to achieve a realization
everyone else appears to have been born with:
that I am nobody but myself."*

RALPH ELLISON

*"Be who you are and say what you feel,
because those who mind don't matter
and those who matter don't mind."*

DR. SEUSS

"You were born an original.
Don't die a copy."

JOHN MASON

STEP FORWARD

I will look for 10 areas of my body to learn to love.

Example:
    I will love my thighs because they remind me of my grandmother's.

1. _____

2. _____

3. _____

4. _____

5. _____

6. _____

7. _____

8. _____

9. _____

10. _____

C ut out and/or photocopy the following page. Frame it and/or make copies of it and post it all over your living space. Whatever you have to do, just remember these words.

Read them every day until you believe them.

10 Steps to Loving Your Body
(No Matter What Size You Are)

by Pat Ballard

1. Never stand in front of a mirror
and think negative thoughts about yourself.

2. Never stand anywhere
and think negative thoughts about yourself.

3. Search carefully for your good points and
when you have found them, nourish them and build on them
and cause them to grow daily.

4. Close your mind to any negative words, thoughts
or actions that someone might send your way.
Don't allow negative thoughts into your subconscious.

5. Always conduct yourself in an honorable fashion
and don't allow your mouth to appear larger than your body.

6. Always do your best to look like you care about yourself,
as no one respects a slob, no matter what size that slob might be.

7. Learn what your best colors are, what your best hair style is,
and what your best clothes style is, and never leave your house
without being dressed accordingly.

8. Always, and without fail, smile and simply say, "Thank you"
when you receive a compliment. Never think or say
that the compliment isn't true.

9. Stop apologizing about your size. Expect everyone to accept you,
respect you, and be happy with you just the way you are.

10. But most of all, you have to love yourself.
When you love yourself, others will love you and respond to you
in the exact manner as you feel about yourself.

I am a unique, one-of-a-kind work of art.
There never has been, and there will never be another me.
I will learn to love the body I have
and will stop trying to force that body
to be or look like something it was
never genetically programmed to be.

About the Author

P at Ballard lives in Nashville, TN. She writes motivational romance novels to show that plus-size women can be just as sexy, romantic and exciting as their slim sisters.

Pat was an active, plump and healthy child growing up as the oldest of six children on a farm between Quitman and Meridian, Mississippi in the 1950s and '60s. She and her siblings perfectly exemplified the roll of genetic dice in terms of body size: Pat and one brother were short and fat, another brother and sister were tall and thin, and a third brother-sister set were average-sized.

All ate the same foods, worked hard and played hard in the days before computer games and 24-hour television programming, and accepted their bodies as their natural birthrights. That is, until Pat discovered height/weight charts when she was 11, followed by fashion and beauty magazines that promoted slimness as the feminine ideal. Both discoveries contributed to a belief that her chubby body was not acceptable as it was. She embarked on a long road of dieting and eating disorders.

By her late teens Pat had so damaged her health by starving herself, purging, and other bulimic behavior that she was suicidal and on the verge of anorexia. With the help of her loving parents she regained her health to some degree, but kept on dieting and trying to shape her body to fit others' ideals.

When Pat was 25 the family moved to East Texas, where she met and married Joe Ballard. When their son, Eric, was three years old, Pat finally quit dieting.

"Life was too short to spend it hungry," she says now. "I needed to have the energy to keep up with an active three-year-old."

She decided to stop trying to lose weight or to keep her body at a specific size. Instead, she would eat as "normally" as she could, exercise when she had time, and what she ended up weighing would just be who she was.

"I came to the conclusion that who I was had nothing to do with my body size," Pat says. "My body was just the package that I was wrapped in. But I made up my mind to learn to love that body, take care of it, and be proud of it."

A new revelation followed: She realized that when she loved and respected herself, others responded to her in the same manner. "The more I accepted myself, held my head up and lived with confidence, the more compliments I received," she says.

She didn't have much support for size acceptance and non-dieting back when she first started fighting against societal messages about "acceptable" weights. Finally, in 1979 a new fashion and beauty magazine emerged that encouraged her attempts to love herself at her natural size: *BBW (Big Beautiful Woman)*. In appreciation for the positive messages *BBW* provided her during an era when size acceptance was practically unheard of, Pat continued subscribing to the magazine until it ceased print publication about 2003.

Outside of (and before) *BBW* magazine, Pat had to rely on her own resources to rebuild her self- and body-esteem.

She initially created her "10 Steps to Loving Your Body" as her personal self-help tool, originally calling them the "10 Commandments of Self-Love."

Pat and her husband and child eventually moved to Nashville so Joe could better pursue his singing/songwriting career. Pat and Joe celebrated their 34th wedding anniversary in early 2008. Eric is now married with two children.

Along the way, Pat found her calling.

She had recognized at an early age that she loved to "make up" and write or tell her own stories. She spent many hours entertaining her younger siblings and cousins with stories she created on the spot, while her audience gathered around her. In school she delighted in English and literature classes, where having to write a short story or poem made her the happiest. The teacher always read her stories aloud to the class.

When Pat was in her mid-teens, she found her literary love—romance novels by Emilie Loring. She knew she wanted to write in the romance genre, but she wanted her books to have a positive effect on as well as entertain her readers. What to write about? Eventually, her own personal struggles pointed the way. After living in her Big Beautiful Body for several years, the proverbial light bulb went off over her head. Of course! Romance novels with Big Beautiful Heroines!

She'd write romance novels where the heroine was large, sexy, and real. Romance novels where the plus-size heroine got her hero just like women do in real life. Romance novels where the heroine would *never* go on a diet to lose weight, but would either love herself from the beginning of the book, or learn to love herself before the book was over.

Pat immediately started writing her novels, and eventually published the first ones with iUniverse.com in 2000. Her husband, Joe, dubbed her "the Queen of Rubenesque Romances"—a title and persona she enjoys playing to the hilt at bookstore and festival appearances.

She began distributing one-page fliers of her "10 Commandments of Self-Love" at the Southern Festival of Books and elsewhere, including her website, www.patballard. com.

Pat noticed at the Southern Festival of Books that people were stopping in their tracks and reading through the "10 Commandments of Self-Love." Tim Segard of iUniverse. com was also watching that response, and told her, "Pat, you know this needs to be a book."

At that moment this book was conceived. Along the way to its birth, the "10 Commandments" morphed into the "10 Steps."

When psychologist and journalist Peggy Elam, Ph.D. founded Pearlsong Press to publish self-affirming and empowering fiction and nonfiction, she acquired rights to Pat's first four novels and her previously unpublished short story collection. *Dangerous Curves Ahead: Short Stories* became Pearlsong Press's inaugural book in May 2004. The republication of *Wanted: One Groom, Nobody's Perfect, His Brother's Child* and *A Worthy Heir* soon followed in trade paperback and ebook format. *Abigail's Revenge* was published in 2005 and *The Best Man* in 2007. *10 Steps to Loving Your Body* is Pat's eighth book.

You can visit Pat on the web at www.patballard.com. Sign up for her free e-mail newsletter, *The Queen's Proclamation*, at www.pearlsong.com/pat_ballard.htm. Look for her other books at your favorite online and offline bookstores, as well as at www.pearlsong.com.

And love your body—no matter what your size!

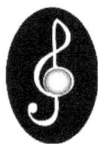

About Pearlsong Press

Pearlsong Press is an independent publishing company dedicated to providing books and resources that entertain while expanding perspectives on the self and the world. The company was founded by Peggy Elam, Ph.D., a psychologist and journalist, in 2003.

Pearls are formed when a piece of sand or grit or other abrasive, annoying, or even dangerous substance enters an oyster and triggers its protective response. The substance is coated with shimmering opalescent nacre ("mother of pearl"), the coats eventually building up to produce a beautiful gem. The self-healing response of the oyster thus transforms suffering into a thing of beauty.

The pearl-creating process reflects our company's desire to move outside a pathological or "disease" based model into a more integrative and transcendent perspective on life, health, and well-being. A move out of suffering into joy. And that, we think, is something to sing about.

Pearlsong Press endorses **Health At Every Size**, an approach to health and well-being that celebrates natural diversity in body size and encourages people to stop focusing on weight (or any external measurement) in favor of listening to and respecting natural appetites for food, drink, sleep, rest, movement, and recreation.

While not every book we publish specifically promotes Health At Every Size, none of our books or other resources will contradict this holistic and body-positive perspective. We encourage you to **enjoy, enlarge, enlighten and enliven yourself** with other Pearlsong Press books, including:

The Program
a novel by Charlie Lovett

*Off Kilter: A Woman's Journey to Peace with Scoliosis,
Her Mother, & Her Polish Heritage*
by Linda C. Wisniewski

Splendid Seniors: Great Lives, Great Deeds
by Jack Adler

The Singing of Swans
a novel about the Divine Feminine
by Mary Saracino

*Beyond Measure:
A Memoir About Short Stature & Inner Growth*
by Ellen Frankel

*Unconventional Means:
The Dream Down Under*
by Anne Richardson Williams

*Taking Up Space:
How Eating Well & Exercising Regularly
Changed My Life*
by Pattie Thomas, Ph.D.
with Carl Wilkerson, M.B.A.
(foreword by Paul Campos,
author of *The Obesity Myth*)

Romance novels and short stories featuring
Big Beautiful Heroines
by Pat Ballard, the Queen of Rubenesque Romances:
The Best Man
Abigail's Revenge
Dangerous Curves Ahead
Wanted: One Groom
Nobody's Perfect
His Brother's Child
A Worthy Heir

& Judy Bagshaw:
At Long Last, Love: A Collection